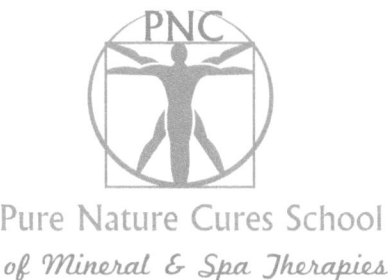

Pure Nature Cures School
of Mineral & Spa Therapies

FIRST AID GUIDE TO MINERALS

Learn how salts, muds, clays, zeolite and diatomaceous earth can save lives in emergencies.

by Galina St George

First Aid Guide to Minerals by Galina St George – Copyright© 2019

TABLE OF CONTENTS

DISCLAIMER

The author of this material sincerely believes that a natural approach to health and maintaining a natural balance within the human body are very important in experiencing energy, vitality, and vibrant health throughout life.

The author recognizes that opinions within scientific and medical fields differ greatly. The purpose of this book is to share educational information and scientific research gathered by the author, scientists, and informed advocates of health and well-being using natural methods and resources.

None of the information contained in this book is intended to diagnose, prevent, treat, or cure any disease, nor is it intended to prescribe any of the techniques, materials or concepts presented as a form of treatment for any illness or medical condition. Before beginning any practice pertaining to procedures described in the book, it is highly recommended that you first obtain the consent and advice of a licensed health care professional.

The information given in this book should be used for educational purposes only, and not as advice or prescription for specific medical conditions. Responsibility for any action taken as a result of reading this book will lie solely with you.

The author assumes no responsibility for the choices you make after your review of the information contained herein and your consultation with a licensed healthcare professional.

If you are on medication, do not start taking or using minerals without your doctor's permission, since being powerful sorbents, clays and zeolite can interfere with medicines.

INTRODUCTION

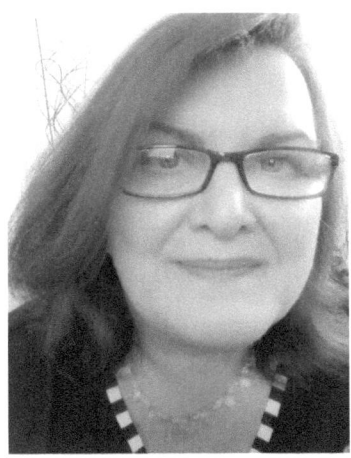

Salts, clays and clay-like minerals have been used both by humans and animals to survive in the harshest conditions as long as they appeared on planet Earth. The reason is that they have always been the most freely and easily available substances to both species.

Animals eat clay instinctively, in order to counteract effects of poisonous substances in plants and to get rid of toxins and internal parasites, as well as to replenish themselves in vital minerals. They roll in mud to rid themselves of ticks, fleas and other skin parasites. They go to salt licks to replenish themselves with minerals.

The use of salts, muds and clays by humans goes back to prehistoric times. People of all cultures were using clays for healing, to prevent food poisoning, heal wounds, stop infections, ulcers, as a source of minerals, to stop hunger pains when food was scarce.

More recently, clays have been used to minimise the effects of radiation in places of radioactive emergencies – such as Chernobyl. Soldiers of Russia and France were given clay rations during World Wars as a means to stop poisoning from dirty water, heal wounds and prevent diarrhoea.

Clays, muds and salts have been used extensively in health and beauty spas to treat chronic health conditions, improve skin and promote rejuvenation. More and more people are beginning to use minerals at home, especially in healing procedures.

This book is a brief guide to those who would like to find out what few people know and talk about – how clays, salts and minerals can help in emergency situations.

Please bear in mind that some of the references in this guide may have expired. I first wrote this guide a few years ago. Still, I had to reference the sources in order to keep in line with the copyright legislation.

Also, I am in the UK and use UK English. Some UK terms have different spelling compared to other English-speaking countries, such as the US. I am letting you know just in case you come across such words.

For the clickable links, pick up the Kindle version of the book free of charge.

Galina St George

Natural Health Practitioner

Treatments & Courses Developer

Blogger

Owner of Pure Nature Cures

School of Mineral & Spa Therapies

www.purenaturecures.com

FIRST AID MINERAL KIT

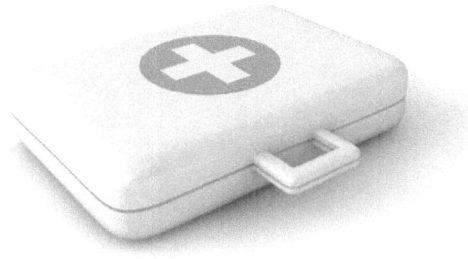

Here is what I suggest you have in your emergency kit at all times:

1. Calcium bentonite or green montmorillonite clay
2. Sodium bentonite clay
3. Magnesium chloride or magnesium sulphate salt
4. Himalayan salt

5. Sodium bicarbonate

6. Zeolite

7. Diatomaceous earth

8. Gauze or any other type of thin cloth (for example, muslin)

9. Cling film or parchment paper

10. Water.

Of course, this is not an exhaustive list. Most people travelling in the wild will have a first aid kit which will include other things, such as scissors etc. Make sure that you have it with you.

CALCIUM BENTONITE CLAY

Calcium Bentonite clay is a natural, mineral clay type substance composed mainly of aluminium, silica, iron oxides, lime, magnesium, and water, in extremely variable proportions, and is generally classified as sedimentary clay. In colour it may be whitish, buff, brown, green, olive, or blue. In colour it may be whitish, buff, brown, green, olive, or blue.

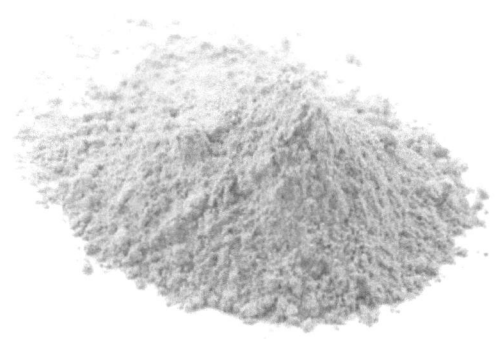

Calcium Bentonite Clay has a very long history of medicinal use in all parts of the world, long before it became known as "bentonite", with remarkable results. Its applications in natural medicine stretch from preventative to curative, dealing with such problems as toxicity, infections, and parasites. Research and use of bentonite clays has shown their strong ability to bind free radicals and heavy metals.

For external applications clays are normally used in compresses, poultices, baths, face masks, body wraps, powder applications to weeping ulcers, nappy rash, weeping eczema, fungal infections.

Clays can also be used as tooth powders – calcium bentonite clays are excellent at removing plaque and whitening teeth, due to their bleaching properties (make sure you don't over-use it for this purpose, since it can be abrasive and can wear down the enamel).

In the cosmetics industry, bentonite clays are used in soaps, toothpastes, face/body packs, and other clay-based products which are beginning to win the consumer over.

GREEN MONTMORILLONITE CLAY

Green montmorillonite clay is one of the most popular and useful clays used in cosmetics and for medicinal purposes.

It contains a variety of minerals and salts including calcium, potassium, dolomite, magnesium, silica, manganese, phosphorous, silicon, copper, and selenium.

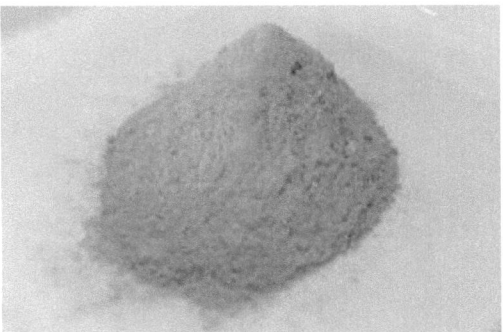

These elements are essential in producing body enzymes which enhance the production of enzymes in all living organisms.

Green Clay – greyish green, the colour is due to the presence of ferrous and magnesium ions. This is the most widely used of the cosmetic and medicinal clays.

Green Montmorillonite Clay is closely related to Bentonite clay – they belong to the same group of smectite clays. Due to its high ionic exchange capacity, it is a superb detoxification product acting like a sponge attracting water and toxins not only to its negatively charged surface, but also inside its numerous canals.

SODIUM BENTONITE CLAY

Sodium Bentonite clay is part of the smectite group of clays. It has a 2:1 structure, expands on hydration (up to 15 times) and has a very high cationic exchange capacity, with sodium being the main exchangeable ion.

It is great clay for treating ulcers, infections and many ailments connected with high acidity, since has powerful alkalising properties. The pH of this clay is very high - normally 9-10 – the highest found in any other clay, and for this reason sodium bentonite clay can be used with great effect for raising body pH as well as detoxification.

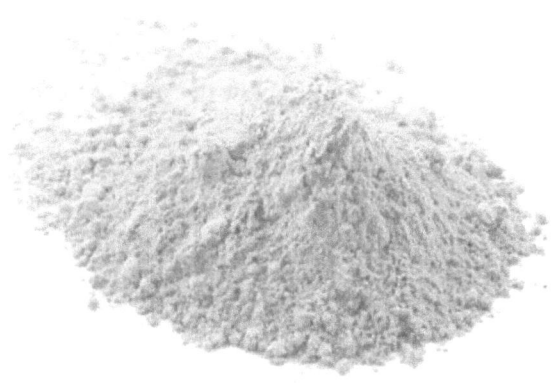

Sodium bentonite expands when hydrated absorbing several times its dry mass in water. This property makes the clay particles expand and increase their negatively charged "active" area many times over. The clay particles become polarised by acquiring a negative charge as a result of hydration.

This negative charge in turn attracts positively-charged ions called "cations" from the environment. This ability of clays is called cation exchange capacity and is an important factor in detoxification processes, since a large majority of toxic substances in our bodies are positively charged. Bentonite clays have the highest CEC among all clays at 70-100.

Because of its high sorptive properties, sodium bentonite clay also works as a magnetic micro-sponge, mopping up what our bodies do not need giving it essential minerals in the process. So this clay works on the body in 3 ways – by exchanging essential to us ions of sodium for heavy metals, absorbing toxic waste, and neutralising body acids, thus raising pH in a very natural way.

MAGNESIUM CHLORIDE & MAGNESIUM SULPHATE SALTS

Magnesium is rightly called a "miracle mineral". There are

few minerals which attract so much attention and instigate so much scientific research. Not only does it participate in over 300 biochemical reactions in the body but also helps maintain many functions, such as steady heart rhythm, normal blood pressure, healthy immune system and strong bones.

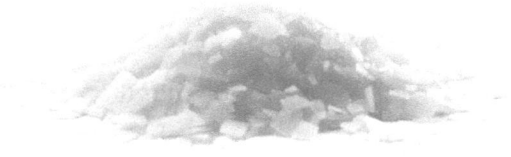

It also helps to maintain the blood sugar at normal levels. It plays a vital role in preventing heart disease, diabetes, cancer, osteoporosis and a whole range of other dangerous and debilitating diseases.

Magnesium is the fourth most abundant mineral in the body. About half of the total body magnesium is found in bones. The other half is found mostly inside cells of body tissues and organs. Only 1% of magnesium is found in the blood where it plays a vital role, so the body works very hard to keep the blood magnesium levels constant.

"...Important participant in enzyme processes which ensure protein biosynthesis and carbohydrate metabolism. It is also very important for the nervous and muscular systems, helps to maintain the healthy tone of the blood vessels. Magnesium is a 'calming' element for the nervous system slowing down the brain activity. It expands the blood vessels and is a natural diuretic. Generally, it is vital for all body systems and processes.

Adult requirement in magnesium is 350-500mg per day. Fresh green vegetables, seafood, soybeans, special nutritional yeasts, seeds, apples and whole grains are rich sources."

https://traceminerals.com/research/magnesium.html

Magnesium has been found to:

- Stimulate protein/fat metabolism
- Reduce inflammation by lowering the levels of histamine and serotonin (mediators of inflammation)
- Strengthen immunity
- Slow down ageing
- Reduce cholesterol levels in the blood
- Reduce blood pressure
- Reduce the effects of stress
- Improve skin condition
- Raise energy levels (magnesium is the essential mineral in the production of energy)
- Promote weight loss.

What happens when we become magnesium-deficient?

Magnesium deficiency is more common than we realise. According to American nutritionists, an average adult needs 200mg more magnesium per day than is obtained from a diet. The fact is, that dietary magnesium is not sufficient in providing the body with this important mineral. Magnesium deficiency can be explained by a number of factors, with main reasons being depletion of soil in minerals.

"Early signs of magnesium deficiency include loss of appetite, nausea, vomiting, fatigue, and weakness. As magnesium deficiency worsens, numbness, tingling, muscle contractions and cramps, seizures, personality changes, abnormal heart rhythms, and coronary spasms can occur." https://ods.od.nih.gov/factsheets/magnesium-HealthProfessional/

Magnesium deficiency may also lead to:

- Loss of energy
- Slowing down of metabolism

- Disturbance in calcium and potassium balance in the blood
- High cholesterol level
- Formation of cholesterol plaque
- Arthritis
- Anxiety
- Depression
- Muscle tension
- Joint pain
- Nervous tension
- Insomnia
- Diabetes.

Both magnesium chloride and sulphate are great, but magnesium chloride is said to be more easily absorbed, since it has smaller molecular weight.

Magnesium chloride comes in flakes and what is called "magnesium oil" – saturated magnesium chloride solution which is oily to touch. Magnesium sulphate, which is also known as Epsom salt, normally comes in fine granules.

HIMALAYAN SALT

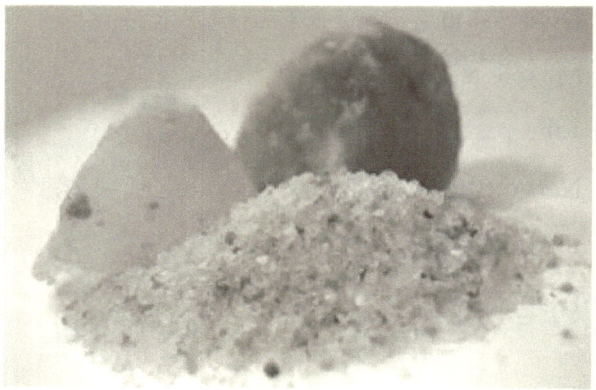

Himalayan Pink Salt is one of the purest salts on Earth, since it is completely free from modern-day pollutants. It was formed as a result of evaporation of ancient seas over 250 million years ago, and contains all the essential elements of the Periodic Table, in perfect balance with each other, as they were found in ancient seas. It is believed that the human body is the mini-ocean as far as its mineral make-up is concerned, so Himalayan salt is one of the best sources of minerals.

Himalayan Pink Salt is one of the purest salts on Earth, since it is completely free from modern-day pollutants. It was formed as a result of evaporation of ancient seas over 250 million years ago, and contains all the essential elements of the Periodic Table, in perfect balance with each other, as they were found in ancient seas. It is believed that the human body is the mini-ocean as far as its mineral make-up is concerned, so Himalayan salt is one of the best sources of minerals.

It is being used in baths and foot baths, to soak tired muscles and relieve fatigue, aches, pains, help with infections of any kind. It is also used as a nose rinse for people suffering from hay fever, as well as sinusitis, and as a mouth wash to help with a sore throat and sore gums.

The salt can also be added to food and drink of sports people, to replenish body salts and rebalance the system. And of course one should not forget those who lose a lot of fluids through sweating or diarrhoea.

Himalayan salt is also used in salt caves to address respiratory problems. Salt lamps are made out of it to promote release of health-boosting ions into the air. And of course one of the major uses of Himalayan salt is as a food product, as a balanced replacement for sodium chloride and sea salt. Of course, like with any salt, one has to watch its intake, and in cases of kidney problems and high blood pressure, intake of any salt has to be closely monitored.

And another, often overlooked, application of this salt is as an additive to animal feed/drinks, especially horses, since they tend to lose a lot of salt during exercise.

Uses:

- Poor circulation

- Poor muscle tone

- Skin infections, acne

- Nail infections

- Tiredness, low energy, general weakness, lethargy

- Sore throat & gums

- Blocked sinuses

- Mineral loss due to excessive & diarrhoea & sweating

- Animals: physical exertion, mineral loss, excessive sweating, diarrhoea.

SODIUM BICARBONATE

Sodium bicarbonate is otherwise known as baking soda. Being one of the most powerful natural cleansers, it has multiple uses in health issues too, due to creating an alkaline environment in the body.

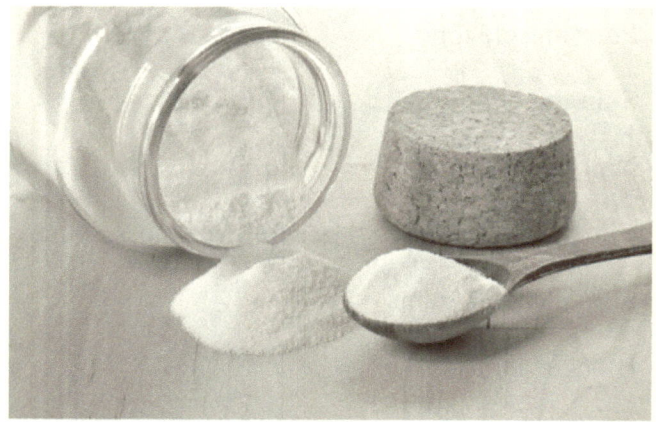

Acidic environment is detrimental to human health, creating beneficial environment for the development of bacterial, viral and fungal infection. Sodium bicarbonate is a cheap and effective way to alkalize the body and remove conditions which lead to disease.

The protective effect of sodium bicarbonate is so strong that it is being used to protect kidneys and other tissues from damaging effects of uranium, mercury, cadmium, arsenic and other heavy metals.

"The oral administration of sodium bicarbonate as a detox cleanse diminishes the severity of the changes produced by uranium in the kidneys. And it does this for all the heavy metals and other toxic chemicals including chemotherapy agents, which are highly lethal even in low dosages.

Since depleted uranium weapons were used starting in the first Gulf War, the United States has polluted the world with uranium oxide and it is showing up more and more in tests doctors perform. With a half-life of several billion years we had better be prepared to get used to dealing with the toxic effects and help our bodies clear it more easily through the kidneys." https://drsircus.com/detox/detox-cleanse/

Dr Sircus recommends using 1-5lbs of sodium bicarbonate in a bath, mixed with 1-5lbs of magnesium chloride flake for stronger effect, to reduce radiation exposure and protect the body from its effects.

He goes on to say: "Clay also should be provided for both internal and external cleansing. The same goes for glutathione suppositories, which should also be taken instantly upon symptom onset, and plenty of spirulina should be on hand and taken regularly. "
https://drsircus.com/detox/detox-cleanse/

So as we can see, sodium bicarbonate, magnesium chloride and clay, used both internally and externally, combined with intake of nutrients such as chlorella and spirulina, are some of the best natural ways to detoxify the body from heavy and radioactive metals.

DIATOMACEOUS EARTH

Diatomaceous Earth, diatomite or DE, is in fact a by-product of simple 2-cell organisms which inhabited the Earth's waters billions of years ago. They were called "diatoms" – hence the name. At the end of their life cycle, the exoskeletons of diatoms formed deposits in various parts of the world, which is what is being mined and used now.

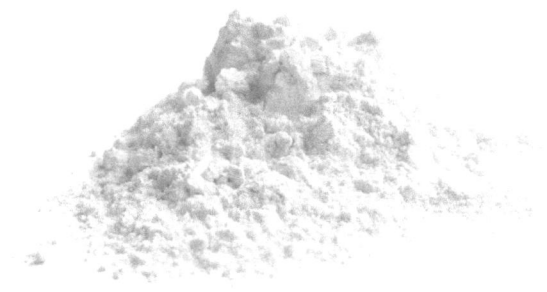

There are two types of diatomaceous earth – fresh water and sea water. Sea water DE is not seen as "clean" compared to the fresh water variety which most people prefer.

Normally, the best diatomaceous earth is white or off-white in colour. The best sources of DE are found in South

America. There may be other great sources too, but I have not come across them yet.

The purity of DE is determined by several factors. One of them is the content of heavy metals. In good quality DE it is extremely low compared to other kinds (for example European).

The other factor is the content of amorphous silica. In good quality DE amorphous silica is close to 100%. In DE of poorer quality, there is a relatively high content of crystalline silica. The danger of crystalline silica is that it is much more aggressive for respiratory organs and more dangerous when inhaled over a period of time.

While it is not a good idea to inhale any DE, the product with a high content of amorphous silica is a lot safer than its counterpart with high crystalline silica content.

While it is harmless to humans and animals, DE is lethal to insects (it destroys their digestive system with its sharp edges), which is why it is so popular in agriculture. It is a safe alternative to insecticide. This is also why many gardeners are turning to DE instead of chemicals.

But of course the insecticide property of diatomite is not confined to gardens and agriculture. Many people use it at home these days, to deal with flea infestation – both in pets and at home. DE is also used against ants, cockroaches, bedbugs and other bugs.

Just think about the misery these creatures cause to us and our pets! And also how using chemicals destroys our immune system and causes so many side effects. This alone will help you stop feeling sorry for the insects that are causing so much misery to us all.

In the garden diatomite is used successfully to get rid of

slugs, snails, caterpillars and other creatures destroying the crops.

And DE is also used to sprinkle on grains, to prevent infestation with all sorts of bugs.

Apart from it all, diatomite is a fantastic sorbent, so can be used for many other things connected with toxins. In fact, in Russia research has found diatomaceous earth to rival zeolite (zeolite wins where heavy metal decontamination is concerned, but DE is close).

The answer is yes for food grade diatomaceous earth. I drink diatomite, to cleanse my body. It makes me feel better in a curious way. My head becomes clearer. I feel more alive, full of energy. A woman I got an email from once wrote how drinking DE helped to stabilise her blood sugar, as well as reduce appetite and weight.

You will of course need to make your own decision. If you

do decide to drink diatomite, look for food grade DE from Peru or Mexico. Make sure that it says 'food grade' on the packaging.

However, we are talking about how to use DE for animals and at home here. If you want to read more about diatomite for human use, read my book "Earth's Humble Healers" (available on Amazon).

First Aid with Minerals

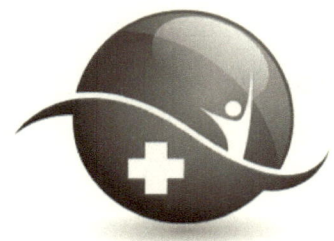

Insect Bites & Skin Infections

Insect bites and skin infections can be painful and uncomfortable. If left untreated, they can get infected. In some cases, an allergy can develop. You should try to seek medical help if at all possible. If it is unavailable, here is what can be done to minimise the pain, discomfort and infection before you can get professional help:

36

1. Mix ½ tsp of sodium bicarbonate and ½ tsp (tea spoonful) of magnesium chloride salt with about 50ml of clean water. Soak a cotton bud or a piece of clean cloth and apply to the area for 15 minutes. Repeat until the inflammation goes down. Applying an ice pack or clean cold object over the area can help relieve the inflammation further.

2. Apply water on the area of the bite and sprinkle some sodium bicarbonate powder on it. Leave on for an hour, wash off and repeat the procedure.

3. If there is no relief as a result of the previous 2 applications, mix 1 tsp of sodium bentonite and 1 part of calcium bentonite clay with warm clean water into a thick paste and apply to the area, covering at least 2 cm beyond the area of the swelling and redness. Apply parchment paper or cling film on the area, wrap up with a bandage (not tight), and leave on for 2-3 hours. Change the poultice for a new one after that. Keep changing until the swelling

and inflammation begins to subside. When the area begins to heal, apply dry clay on it (no bandage).

MINOR BURNS

In cases of burns it is important to make sure that the area gets cooled down as soon as possible. Always follow a 1st aid procedure to minimise the damage from a burn.

Normally it would be advised to keep cooling the area under running cold water for 15 minutes, or until the pain has subsided. Not only this reduces the pain, but also further tissue damage.

Once the area is cooled down, some sources advise on applying sodium bicarbonate powder to the area to minimise the damage. Lavender essential oil is claimed to have profound healing effect on burns when applied as it is, as often as required.

Another type of application would involve a cold clay

compress. Mix very cold water with 1 part of sodium bentonite and 1 part of calcium bentonite clay to make a paste. Apply to the area in a thin layer, cover with a piece of parchment paper or cling film. Wrap it up with a thin layer of gauze. Apply an ice pack on top of it (if available).

Wash off the poultice in about 2 hours, repeat the initial procedure after this. This kind of treatment is only suitable for minor burns. For more serious burns, follow first aid instructions and seek medical help as soon as possible.

THROAT & MOUTH INFECTIONS

1. A very well-known remedy for sore throat and mouth infections includes the use of salt, sodium bicarbonate and water. Add 1 tsp of Himalayan salt, 1 tsp of sodium bicarbonate to 1 glass of warm boiled water. Mix it well and gargle or rinse the mouth as frequently as possible.

2. Add 1 tsp of calcium bentonite clay and 1 tsp of magnesium chloride flakes to 1 glass of warm water. Let it

stand for 15 minutes before using. Gargle or rinse the mouth with the mixture as often as required.

BLOCKED NOSE

Make a 1% solution of Himalayan salt with water. To prepare it, take ¼ of a teaspoonful of Himalayan salt (approximately 1g), and mix it with 100ml of water. Use a pipette or a tea spoon to put a few drops (5-6) of the solution into each nostril.

If you have a syringe, it's even better. Wait for 1 minute and then blow your nose one nostril at a time. This procedure can be repeated every 2 hours where the blockage is heavy and there is feeling that the sinuses may be congested as well.

DIARRHOEA

Diarrhoea should always be treated medically where possible, since it is a dangerous condition which may have multiple causes, and if left untreated, can lead to dehydration and even death. The following recipe is for cases where there is no possibility to get medical help quickly (emergency cases, such as "lost in a jungle", war situations, or being in a country where immediate medical help is unavailable).

Proper hydration is crucial in cases of diarrhoea. In medical conditions, a saline drink would be given, or a saline drip in cases of extreme dehydration. In non-medical emergency conditions, salt needs to be added to clean (boiled) water (preferably Himalayan, but if it is not available, any sodium containing salt will do – such as sea salt or table salt). Add ½ tsp to 550ml of water (about 1 pint).

During both World Wars, clays were used to stop diarrhoea. Zeolite is another substance which is used in some countries (Japan, Cuba) to make anti-diarrhoea medications.

In extreme circumstances where there is no medical help

available, mix 1 table spoonful of calcium bentonite clay and 1 table spoonful of zeolite clinoptilolite powder with 450ml of water. Drink on an empty stomach, 1 glass every 2 hours. Ensure that the clay and zeolite particles are suspended in water, since this will provide the best effect.

FOOD POISONING

Clays and zeolite are excellent sorbents. This means that they can absorb toxins created by the bacteria which cause food poisoning. This property has long been used both by humans and animals to neutralise poisons from foods which may have toxins in them, and as a remedy against food poisoning. As I have already mentioned, clay used to be part of the rations issued to Russian and French soldiers during WWI.

The drink to counteract damaging effects of food poisoning would be similar to the one for diarrhoea. Mix 1 table spoonful of calcium bentonite clay and 1 table spoonful of zeolite clinoptilolite powder with 550ml of water. Drink it on an empty stomach, 1 glass every hour. Ensure that clay and zeolite particles are suspended in water, since this will provide the best effect.

The effect of clay in such cases may be explained by clay particles not only absorbing the toxins created by bacteria, but also by enveloping bacteria in the stomach and intestines and depriving it of food sources. However, this is only a theory which I haven't seen scientific proof to yet.

WATER FILTRATION IN EXTREME CONDITIONS

Clay and zeolite can be used to filter water. In fact, zeolite is routinely used for this purpose by water companies.

To prepare a water filter in extreme conditions, use a clean cloth, spread clay and zeolite (or just zeolite) over it – about 10cm thick, pull the sides together to make a sack, flatten the bag with the minerals over a hard mesh and pour water through it. This will remove major impurities, but you will still need to boil water to eliminate bacteria and parasites.

Another way is to simply put clay and zeolite in the water and mix it well. Let the particles settle, mix again. The water at the top of the particles can be strained and boiled for use.

HEAVY METAL & RADIATION EXPOSURE

In the large majority of cases, heavy metals and radiation have a damaging effect on the body over a long period of time – except in cases of emergency where there has been a major incident or you have got into an area of severe contamination.

Most of us are routinely exposed to heavy metals coming from car fumes, industrial fumes, cigarettes, plastics, water, some foods, medicines, pesticides, old paint and other sources.

Fast and acute exposure often leads to heavy metal poisoning and radiation disease. Such cases are considered an emergency and must always be addressed in a hospital environment since procrastination may lead to internal organ and brain damage, and in severe cases – death. In cases of acute radioactive exposure, damage to health can be devastating and irreversible.

Both clay and zeolite are excellent sorbents for heavy metals and free radicals which form as a result of radioactive exposure.

Of course, medical treatment would involve a number of procedures aimed at chelating heavy metals and removing free radicals out of the body.

In an emergency, clay and zeolite are often used to minimise the first impact of heavy metal and radioactive exposure. They act like scavengers, mopping up heavy metals and free radicals and taking them out of the body.

Zeolite and clay are not only used to bury nuclear reactors in emergency situations, but are also given to people and animals to protect them from the main damage in the first few days of exposure to radiation. Biscuits with zeolite were given to people in the Chernobyl area during the nuclear accident, to promote decontamination.

A drink with clay and zeolite would be prepared the following way: 1 tbsp (table spoonful) of clay, 1 tbsp of zeolite mixed with 550 ml of water. This can be taken every hour, preferably on an empty stomach.

WOUNDS, ULCERS & GANGRENE

Wounds can become infected in extreme conditions. Sometimes they can lead to ulcers, and even gangrene. In normal conditions medical help is of utmost importance. However, in extreme conditions it may not be forthcoming for some time.

Clays have been used by humans to stop a wound from

getting infected, or even to stop an infection, development of ulcers and even gangrene in some cases. I am speaking about extreme cases where antibiotics would not be available.

There is great evidence of French doctors treating Buruli flesh-eating ulcers in African countries using green clay applications. They simply mix green clay with water and apply on the area of an ulcer or infection. Healing results have been remarkable.

There is also information about MRSA bacteria which is resistant to common antibiotics being destroyed by green clay. https://nsf.gov/discoveries/disc_summ.jsp

The explanations are multiple, but the fact is that clay applications have saved many people's lives.

MUSCLE SPRAIN

Muscle sprains are normally treated with cold pack

applications. I am not going to add anything to this. Cold works best in acute tissue injuries.

However, as time passes, 2-3 days after the injury happened, it is important to ensure that tissues are healing without forming lesions and subsequent lumps which may become painful and limit movements of extremities.

So in such cases warm magnesium chloride or magnesium sulphate (Epsom salt) compresses are applied to the area.

Here is how to prepare such a compress:

Add 1 tbsp of salt to very warm water (about 100ml). Soak a piece of cloth. Apply on the affected area. Wrap it up with cling film and a warm scarf. Leave on for 2-3 hours, or even overnight. Repeat as necessary.

MUSCLE SPASM (CRAMP)

Muscle spasms normally happen when there is insufficient

magnesium in the body, or in cases of dehydration and water/ salt imbalance. It is important to realise what the underlying reason is before beginning to treat it.

Magnesium salt applications over the body help really well in cases of muscle spasms. Mix 1 part of magnesium salt (magnesium chloride is best, but magnesium sulphate is good too) with 1 part of water. Spread it over the body by hand, paying special attention to the areas which are most affected by cramps. Repeat twice a day or as frequently as required.

JOINT PAIN

As we age, our joints become less mobile. Sometimes they become inflamed causing considerable pain and discomfort to a person. Warm magnesium compresses are the best solution for such cases.

There are 2 recipes I would like to share here:

1. Add 1 tbsp of salt to very warm water (about 100ml). Soak a piece of cloth. Apply on the affected area. Wrap it up with cling film and a warm scarf. Leave on for 2-3 hours, or even overnight. Repeat as necessary.

2. Clay and magnesium compress: mix 2 parts of green montmorillonite clay with 1 part of magnesium and 3 parts of water (or more – depending on the consistency you want to get). Apply the paste on an affected joint, wrap it up with cling film and a warm scarf. Leave it on overnight or at least for 2 hours. This can be repeated 2-3 times a day, or as required.

BLUNT OBJECT INJURY

These injuries normally happen when we are hit with a blunt object or when we run into something (or someone). Normally such injuries result in internal haemorrhage leading to bruising.

It is very difficult to stop the bruising completely.

However, it is still possible to minimise it and bring relief to the area at the same time. A cold clay compress can do wonders for such injuries.

Mix one part of clay (calcium bentonite or green montmorillonite) with cold water to a paste. Apply on the area. Apply parchment paper or cling film and a piece of cloth. Apply an ice pack over the injury. Leave it on for 5-10 minutes, remove for 15 minutes.

Repeat the procedure for 1-2 hours. Make sure that you take the ice pack off repeatedly to make sure that the tissues don't get damaged. If you don't have access to ice, use cold water or any cold object.

PARASITE INFESTATION

If you are out and about in the wild for a long period of time, especially in warmer climates or in places where access to clean water is limited, the risk of parasite infestation becomes real.

51

Of course, dirty water is not the only culprit. Food can also become infected with parasites. And there is a risk of getting bitten by parasite-spreading insects.

If you suspect that you have been infected, seek medical help as soon as you can. In the meantime, taking 1-2 heaped teaspoonfuls of diatomaceous earth mixed with a glass of clean water 3-4 times daily could help to prevent further infestation and eliminate at least some of the parasites from the system.

Animals (dogs, cats, horses) can also be given DE – about 1 teaspoonful mixed with food or water for smaller animals and 5-6 table spoonfuls mixed with water or food for larger animals 3-4 times a day.

CONCLUSION

Minerals are very versatile substances. There are many varieties of clays, salts and other minerals in nature, all with their own unique properties. I have described only some of them, so that if you ever find yourself in a situation where what nature has to offer is the only solution, you will know how to use what you have at hand.

Since clays and salts are not always freely available everywhere you go, it is best to stock up and have them with you if you intend to use them as first aid remedies.

If you are on medication, minerals such as clay and zeolite need to be taken 2-3 hours after taking medicines since they are powerful sorbents. It is important to seek your doctor's advice if you decide to start taking clay, zeolite or diatomaceous earth while undergoing medical treatment.

FURTHER INFORMATION & LINKS

More information about salts, clays and minerals can be found in the following books:

1. Earth's Humble Healers

Learn how to use salts, muds and clays for better health, youth & vitality. Plus 80 health & beauty recipes.

2. How Clays Work

Science & application of clays and clay-like minerals in health & beauty.

3. Magnesium at Home

25 Most Common Health Conditions & How Magnesium Salts Can Help.

4. Mineral Healing Recipe Book

Practical and Easy to Follow Guide Describing How to Use Salts, Muds, Clays, Zeolite and Diatomaceous Earth for Health and Beauty Purposes at Home and in Clinics

All of these books are available on Amazon.

COURSES

Are you a Natural Health or Beauty Practitioner, and would like to get qualified as a Mineral & Spa Therapist, to be able to offer mineral-based treatments to your clients? Or perhaps you are simply interested in natural health remedies and treatments and would like to find out more about minerals? Take a look at the courses we have to offer and see if any of them would be of interest to you –

courses.purenaturecures.com

For more information about minerals and to read my latest blog posts, check out my site https://purenaturecures.com

If you are interested in learning more about magnesium and its health benefits, check out my magnesium blog – https://magnesiumoil.org.uk.

GET IN TOUCH

If you have any questions after reading this book, please get in touch with me at galina@purenaturecures.com.

NOTES